1

Table of Contents

How to help your ADHD child manage symptoms of anxiety

The ADHD-Anxiety Connection

What an Anxious Child With ADHD May Look Like

Why Anxiety Is Sometimes Misdiagnosed as ADHD

ADHD Adults

STRESS & ANXIETY

A woman with ADHD showing signs of anxiety

Can Untreated ADD Cause Anxiety?

Treatment for the Symptoms of Anxiety Disorders

What to Expect From ADHD and Anxiety

How to Treat ADHD and Anxiety

How to treat kids with anxiety and ADHD

Medication dosing for children with ADHD

Treating both anxiety and ADHD

Therapy and relaxation techniques

INTRODUCTION

Rates of anxiety in the presence of ADHD in the general population range from 13 to 50%, and these co-morbidities together are associated with greater risk of long term impairments than children with either condition. However, only a few studies have examined the frequency or the clinical impact of anxiety in children with ADHD. It was found that individuals with ADHD had higher frequency of anxiety, Since having ADHD is already known to negatively effect functioning, it is assumed that having anxiety in addition to ADHD will have additive negative impact on children.

In light of this, it is possible that the clinical presentation in ADHD would not be worsened by having anxiety symptoms. Therefore, is it important to further investigate the contribution of having anxiety symptoms in co-morbid ADHD on various aspects of the clinical presentation.

ADHD

Attention deficit hyperactive disorder, or ADHD, is a condition characterized by inattention, hyperactivity, impulsiveness, or a combination. About 60 percent of children with ADHD in the United States become adults with ADHD; that's about 4 percent of the adult population, or 8 million adults. Less than 20 percent of adults with ADHD have been diagnosed or treated, and only about one-quarter of those adults seek help.

Thought to be biological and most often genetic, ADHD takes place very early in brain development. Adults with ADHD may exhibit the same symptoms they had as children, and although hyperactivity often diminishes by adulthood, inattentiveness and impulsivity may persist.

Symptoms

ADHD symptoms often include an inability to focus, disorganization, and restlessness. Adults with ADHD may have a hard time organizing things, listening to instructions, remembering details, or difficulty completing tasks, which can affect their relationships at home, school, and work. People who have ADHD may exhibit different symptoms, and they may experience them at different levels of severity, ranging from mild to significant impairment.

ADHD and mental health disorders

Adults with ADHD are likely to have an anxiety disorder, depression, bipolar disorder, or other comorbid psychiatric disorder. (The term "comorbid" refers to a condition that exists with another.)

About 50 percent of adults with ADHD also suffer from an anxiety disorder. Adult ADHD symptoms that coexist with an anxiety disorder or other disorders may significantly impair the ability to function.

Diagnosis

Proper diagnosis relies on a comprehensive clinical evaluation by a health professional, who will take into account personal history, self-reported symptoms, and mental-status testing, as well as early development problems and symptoms of inattention, distractibility, impulsivity, and emotional instability.

Overlapping symptoms of comorbid psychiatric conditions often complicate getting an accurate diagnosis.

A health professional will ask questions like these during a consultation:

- Do your behaviors and feelings show that you have problems with attention and hyperactivity?
- Do you have a hard time keeping your temper or staying in a good mood?

- Do these problems happen to you at work and at home?
- Do family members and friends see that you have these problems?
- Have you had these problems since you were a child?
- Do you have any physical or mental health problems that might affect your behavior?

Treatment

Medication is a cornerstone of treatment for adults with ADHD. Research has shown that stimulants and some non stimulants can improve the symptoms of ADHD, helping people pay attention, concentrate, and control their impulses.

Most people also benefit from behavioral, psychological, educational, and coaching interventions. A helpful resource for locating support groups or professionals with appropriate expertise is CHADD (Children and Adults with Attention Deficit Hyperactivity Disorder).

Anxiety disorders and other comorbid conditions may come about as a result of living with ADHD. Having a comorbid anxiety disorder can make treatment more complicated. A health professional will define the areas of impairment (such as problems relating to attention or impulsivity at work or school, sleeping, or family life) and help select the most favorable treatment option.

In addition to prescribing medication for ADHD, a health professional may recommend CBT (cognitive-behavior therapy) for comorbid anxiety. Some stimulant-drug treatments for ADHD may worsen anxiety symptoms in patients with comorbid anxiety disorders.

A health professional should focus on the disorder associated with the highest degree of impairment. If ADHD is the cause of anxiety, treating the ADHD may reduce the anxiety. If anxiety is independent of ADHD, however, a doctor will determine the proper medication. One health professional may decide to treat the anxiety first; another may treat both conditions simultaneously.

Myths About ADHD

Myth 1: ADHD Is Not a Real Disorder

ADHD is recognized as a disorder/disability by the Centers for Disease Control, the National Institutes of Health, the United States Congress, the Department of Education, the Office for Civil Rights, the American Medical Association, and every other major professional medical, psychiatric, psychological and educational association or organization. Part of the misunderstanding about ADHD stems from the fact that no specific test can definitively identify ADHD. A doctor cannot confirm the diagnosis through laboratory tests as they can other medical diseases such as diabetes. Though there is not yet a specific medical test for diagnosing ADHD, clear and specific criteria must be met for a diagnosis to be made. Using these criteria and an in-depth history and detailed information about behaviors, a reliable diagnosis can be made. An additional misconception may occur because symptoms of ADHD may not always seem clear-cut. We all experience problems with attention and focus to some degree. For an individual with ADHD, however, these symptoms are so severe that they impair daily functioning. ADHD represents an extreme on a continuum of behaviors. Sometimes the behaviors are misunderstood. Symptoms of ADHD can certainly appear similar to other conditions. That is why the health professional making the diagnosis must first rule out any other pre-existing conditions or causes for the symptoms.

Myth 2: ADHD Is Caused by Poor Parenting

This myth has often created negative feelings of self blame in parents of children with ADHD. It is simply not true that poor parenting causes ADHD. What is true, however, is that positive parenting with clear and consistent expectations and consequences and a home environment with predictable routines can help manage symptoms of ADHD. Conversely, a home setting that is chaotic or parenting that is punitive and critical can worsen symptoms of ADHD.

Myth 3: Only Children Can Have ADHD

Though the symptoms of ADHD must be present by age 7 in order to meet the criteria for diagnosis, many individuals remain undiagnosed until adulthood. For some adults, a diagnosis is made after their own child is diagnosed. As the adult learns more and more about ADHD, he or she recognizes the ADHD traits in themselves. They may think back to their own childhood and recall the struggles in school and problems with attention that were never treated. It is often a huge relief to finally understand and put a name to the condition causing the problems. Thirty percent to 70 percent of children with ADHD continue to exhibit symptoms into adulthood. Often times, the hyperactive behaviors common with children decrease with age, but symptoms of restlessness, distractibility, and inattention continue. Left untreated adult ADHD can create chronic difficulties with work and in relationships and can result in secondary issues such as anxiety, depression and substance abuse.

Myth 4: You Have to Be Hyperactive to Have ADHD

This myth has lead to a lot of confusion about ADHD. Even the name of the condition itself -– Attention Deficit Hyperactivity Disorder -– leads to misunderstanding. There are actually three different types of ADHD: the predominately hyperactive-impulsive type, the predominately inattentive type, and the combined type. The predominately inattentive type does not include symptoms of hyperactivity at all. Because of this, it is often referred to simply as ADD. An individual with the inattentive symptoms may present as daydreamy and easily distracted, disorganized, forgetful, careless. The predominately inattentive type of ADHD is much less disruptive to others around the individual. So it often gets overlooked, but it is no less stressful for the individual. It is also important to point out that adults with ADHD may lose some of the hyperactive behaviors that may have been present in childhood. Instead the hyperactivity is replaced with a sense of restlessness. Click on ADD verses ADHD to read more.

Myth 5: Use of Stimulant Medications Leads to Drug Abuse and Addictions

Research has actually found the opposite result. If left untreated, individuals with ADHD are at a higher risk of substance abuse. This is likely because secondary problems (such as anxiety or depression) develop from the untreated ADHD and the individual uses the illicit substances to help relieve the ADHD symptoms. It becomes a way of self medicating, though it is obviously not effective. For those who receive appropriate treatment, which often does include stimulant medications, the rate of substance abuse is much lower.

Myth 6: If You Can Keep Focused on Some Activities, You Do Not Have ADHD

It can be quite confusing to see someone with ADHD focus intently on an activity when ADHD seems to be an "attention deficit." It is actually more appropriate to describe ADHD as a condition in which individuals have difficulty regulating their attention. Though they may have extreme problems focusing, organizing, and completing certain mundane tasks, they are often able to focus intently on other activities that interest and engage them. This tendency to become absorbed in tasks that are stimulating and rewarding is called hyperfocus.

Myth 7: Medication Can Cure ADHD

Medications do not cure ADHD rather they help to control symptoms of ADHD on the day they are taken. ADHD is a chronic condition that does not go away, though symptoms may change or lessen over time. Many individuals develop coping and organizing strategies to help manage and control symptoms over their lifetime. Some individuals continue to need medical treatment through medications to help control their symptoms into adulthood.

Myth 8: ADHD is Over-Diagnosed

ADHD AND ANXIETY

An estimated 264 million people worldwide have an anxiety disorder. Our World Data

An estimated 31.1% of U.S. adults experience any anxiety disorder at some time in their lives. National Institute of Mental Health

An estimated 19.1% of U.S. adults had any anxiety disorder in the past year. National Institute of Mental Health

Anxiety is one of the most common forms of mental illness. Anxiety can affect your health. If you suffer from an anxiety disorder, research suggests that you may run a higher risk of experiencing physical health problems, too. So when you manage your anxiety, you're also taking care of your physical health.

Most people who seek treatment experience significant improvement and enjoy an improved quality of life. Find a Therapist.

Whether you have everyday stress, everyday anxiety or an anxiety disorder you can learn important strategies to help you manage and move forward.

Exercising, good nutrition, adequate sleep, and trying to reduce stress all contribute to your well-being.

Relationship between ADHD and Anxiety

The link between ADHD and anxiety

If you've been diagnosed with attention deficit hyperactivity disorder (ADHD), you may also have another mental health disorder. Sometimes symptoms of other conditions can be masked by the symptoms of ADHD. It's estimated that over 60 percent of people with ADHD have a comorbid, or coexisting, condition.

Anxiety is one condition that is often seen in people with ADHD. About 50 percent of adults and up to 30 percent of children with ADHD also have an anxiety disorder. Keep reading to learn more about the connection between these two conditions.

If you have ADHD, it may be difficult to recognize the symptoms of anxiety. ADHD is an ongoing condition that often starts in childhood and can continue into adulthood. It can affect your ability to concentrate, and may result in behavioral problems, such as:

• hyperactivity

• lack of attention

• lack of impulse control

• fidgeting and trouble sitting still

• difficulty organizing and completing tasks

An anxiety disorder is more than just feeling occasionally anxious. It's a mental illness that is serious and long lasting. It can make you feel distressed, uneasy, and excessively frightened in benign, or regular, situations. If you have an anxiety disorder, your symptoms may be so severe that they affect your ability to work, study, enjoy relationships, or otherwise go about your daily activities.

The symptoms of ADHD are slightly different from those of anxiety. ADHD symptoms primarily involve issues with focus and concentration. Anxiety symptoms, on the other hand, involve issues with nervousness and fear.

ADHD symptoms and Anxiety symptoms

- difficulty concentrating or paying attention
- trouble completing tasks
- forgetfulness
- inability to relax or feelings of restlessness
- difficulty listening to and following instructions
- inability to focus for long periods of time
- chronic feelings of worry or nervousness
- fear without an obvious cause
- irritability
- trouble sleeping or insomnia
- headaches and stomachaches
- fear of trying new things

Even though each condition has unique symptoms, sometimes the two conditions mirror each other. That can make it difficult to tell whether you have ADHD, anxiety, or both.

How can you tell the difference

Though a professional evaluation is necessary, family members may be able to tell the difference between ADHD and anxiety. The key is to watch how your symptoms present over time.

If you have anxiety, you may be unable to concentrate in situations that cause you to feel anxious. On the other hand, if you have ADHD, you'll find it difficult to concentrate most of the time, in any type of situation.

If you have both ADHD and anxiety, the symptoms of both conditions may seem more extreme. For example, anxiety can make it even more difficult for someone with ADHD to pay attention and follow through on tasks.

Understanding comorbidity

It's not clear why there's a connection between ADHD and anxiety, and doctors don't fully understand what causes either condition. Genetics may be responsible for both conditions, and may also cause comorbidity. Researchers have also observed several other conditions that are commonly seen alongside ADHD, including:

- anxiety
- depression
- autism
- sleep disorders
- dyslexia
- substance abuse
- bipolar disorder

Possible causes for ADHD include genetics, environmental toxins, or premature birth. It's possible that these causes could also contribute to anxiety.

Treatment

Treating ADHD and anxiety simultaneously may be challenging because some medications for ADHD can exacerbate anxiety symptoms. Both conditions need to be treated, though. Your doctor may choose to focus first on the condition that's the most disruptive to your quality of life. They may also provide suggestions for ways to manage the other condition.

The treatments your doctor may recommend for both ADHD and anxiety include:

cognitive and behavioral therapy

relaxation techniques

meditation

prescription medication

It's important to be truthful and open with your doctor about your symptoms. This is especially true if you suspect you're experiencing two conditions simultaneously. Your doctor will want to know if a treatment is making one or both of your conditions worse. That will help them tailor your treatment.

Outlook

If you have ADHD, it's important to tell your doctor about all of your symptoms, even if you think they're unrelated. It's possible you could have an additional condition, such as anxiety. You should also let your doctor know about any new symptoms, as you could develop anxiety or another condition over time.

Once your doctor has diagnosed you with both ADHD and anxiety, you'll be able to begin treatment for both conditions.

Managing your anxiety

An anxiety disorder is a mental condition that needs to be treated by a mental health professional. There are things you can do, though, to try to reduce your symptoms.

Learn your triggers

In some people, anxiety may be triggered by specific events, like speaking in public or calling someone on the phone. Once you've identified your triggers, work with your doctor to help come up with ways to manage your anxiety in these situations. For example, preparing notes and practicing a presentation may help you feel less anxious when speaking in front of others.

Get seven to eight hours of sleep every night

Being tired may trigger anxiety or increase your risk for feeling anxious. Try to sleep for seven to eight hours every night. If you're having trouble falling asleep, try meditating or taking a warm bath before bed to help quiet your mind. Also plan to go to sleep and wake up at the same time every day. Setting a sleep schedule can be an effective way to train your body to sleep

Anxiety in Adults With ADHD

Many adults with attention deficit hyperactivity disorder (ADHD) also struggle with anxiety that impairs their lives. Sometimes this anxiety develops as a result of the ADHD symptoms.

Symptoms of Chronic Anxiety

If you have difficulty managing the everyday demands of life, are chronically late, forgetful, have trouble meeting deadlines and obligations, become overwhelmed with finances, tune out in conversations, speak or act impulsively, lack tact in social situations—then certainly this can bring about feelings of chronic anxiety.

You may worry about keeping track of it all. You may worry about what will go wrong next. When will the next "let down" occur? What will I say next to embarrass myself or someone else? You may dread that next time when you are rushing to an important appointment that you will surely be late to again.

Sometimes adults with ADHD also worry in a different way. It can be so difficult to manage daily activities that you may find yourself experiencing anxiety in a pressured way as you try to organize yourself.

Do these concerns sound familiar? "I must remember to turn in the contract by Feb. 1"; "The report has to be finished by Monday"; and "I cannot forget to pick up the kids early from school Friday because they have a dentist appointment."

In these situations, your mind may get fixated on worry. For some people, this is a helpful way to organize and remember. For others, this self-imposed pressure becomes even more debilitating. With such enormous worry and burden hanging over your head, you may find that you shut down even more. Some people even experience a sense of paralysis that prevents them from moving forward at all.

ADHD and Anxiety Disorders

In addition to the anxiety symptoms associated with ADHD described above, research does find a strong association between ADHD and anxiety disorders.

Approximately 25 percent to 40 percent of adults with ADHD also have an anxiety disorder.

Anxiety disorders can manifest themselves in a variety of physical, mood, cognitive and behavioral symptom patterns. Common features of these disorders are excessive anxiety, worry, nervousness, and fear. This is often accompanied by feelings of restlessness, being "keyed up" or constantly on edge, problems with concentration (or mind going blank), sleep disturbances, muscle tension, irritability, fatigue, and feeling overwhelmed.

It can be very difficult to relax and participate fully in life with these impairing symptoms. The person quickly begins to avoid situations in which a negative outcome could occur. If that person is able to face these situations, he or she may only be able to do so by spending excessive time and effort preparing. The anxiety can result in procrastination in behavior or decision-making and the need to repeatedly seek reassurances due to worries.

An Overview of Generalized Anxiety Disorder

Treatment

It is clear that features of ADHD inattention, restlessness, procrastination, sleep problems, feeling overwhelmed can overlap with symptoms of anxiety. So one of the first steps in planning treatment is to decipher whether these impairments are coming from the ADHD (secondary to the ADHD) or whether they are the result of a separate, co-existing anxiety disorder.

Whether or not a person meets the diagnostic criteria for an anxiety disorder, it is clear that symptoms of ADHD can result in chronic anxiety that can further impair a person's functioning, happiness, and level of self-esteem. It is important to understand and manage the full spectrum of ADHD. Many adults with ADHD and anxiety benefit from cognitive behavioral therapy in combination with appropriate medical treatment.

ADHD & Anxiety in Children

It's common for children diagnosed with Attention Deficit Hyperactivity Disorder (ADHD) to struggle with anxiety, whether it's a few symptoms or a full-blown disorder. The Centers for Disease Control and Prevention (CDC) estimates that up to 30% of children with ADHD also have an anxiety disorder,[1] and a review of the current research shows comorbidity between ADHD and anxiety reaching 25% in many samples.

Some of the symptoms of ADHD, such as frequent interrupting, blurting out, fidgeting, and forgetfulness, can be very intrusive and increase stress levels for children. If children are consistently reprimanded for talking out of turn in school, for example, they are likely to experience higher stress and low self-esteem. Many children diagnosed with ADHD struggle with working memory, time-management skills, and organizational skills. This can make it difficult to follow daily routines and complete short- and long-term tasks. It can also result in chronic stress.

Children with ADHD also struggle with emotional regulation. ADHD often causes kids to become flooded with emotions, positive or negative, which can be difficult to manage in the moment. If a child is flooded with feelings of anxiety, for example, that child might struggle to make sense of his thoughts and become caught in a cycle of negative and anxious thinking.

One of our 3-minute Self-Assessments may help identify if you or your child could benefit from further diagnosis and treatment.

Difficulty regulating emotions and coping with anxious thoughts can manifest in different ways for different kids. While some kids might completely check out and turn their anxious thoughts inward, others are likely to act out with negative behaviors. Tuning into your child's baseline behaviors will help you assess for co-existing anxiety when notice a shift in behaviors.

Symptoms of anxiety in children:
- sleep disturbance (difficulty falling or staying asleep)
- increased irritability
- argumentative
- withdraws from peers
- school refusal
- clowning around in school

- hair twirling, skin picking, or other anxious behaviors.

Anxiety symptoms can mimic ADHD symptoms

Misdiagnosis can and does occur when it comes to children with ADHD and/or anxiety. The best course of action to ensure an accurate diagnosis is a thorough evaluation by a neuropsychologist.

Anxiety looks a lot like ADHD for many children, so it's important to have your child evaluated to determine the best course of treatment.

The following are just a few of the many ways in which symptoms of ADHD and anxiety overlap:

Inattention: An anxious child might check out and tune into his worries. To the teacher or parent, this looks like inattention. For an ADHD child, inattention is a symptom of the disorder.

Poor peer relationships: A child with social anxiety will struggle to make and maintain friendships due to fears about rejection or difficulty regulating emotional thoughts while engaged with peers. A child with ADHD is likely to have low impulse control and poor social skills, which makes it difficult to sustain friendships.

Slow work habits: Anxious children can struggle with perfectionism, making it difficult to complete in-class and homework assignments. An ADHD child struggles with the workload due to poor organizational skills and reduced attention span.

Constant movement: Anxious children tend to move around a lot (foot tapping, tipping chair) and ask constant questions in an attempt to manage anxious energy. ADHD kids fidget because of low impulse control.

While there are symptoms that overlap, it's important to note that anxious children display more perfectionist behaviors and worry about socializing with others, while ADHD kids struggle with impulse control and organization. A complete neuropsychological evaluation, including at least one classroom evaluation, will help determine whether a child's behaviors are rooted in ADHD, anxiety, or some combination of the two.

How to help your ADHD child manage symptoms of anxiety

Keep a trigger tracker:

Understanding what particular stressors cause the most anxiety for your child helps your child learn to predict anxiety-inducing situations and manage symptoms as they arise. If test anxiety triggers distorted thinking, for example, your child can meet with the classroom teacher to determine test-taking strategies that might help in the moment.

Your child can keep a "worry thermometer" in his backpack or desk to jot times when he felt "hot" with anxiety during the school day. He can color in the thermometer to the appropriate level and write down the time of day. This will help the classroom teacher understand his anxiety hot s pots. Kids can also use the worry thermometer at home, or use a worry journal to keep a list of anxious and intrusive thoughts.

Teach thought stopping:

Anxious kids struggle with flooding. Anxious thoughts tend to overwhelm kids all at once, and it can be difficult to recover once the brain shifts into a pattern of anxious thinking.

Teach your child to practice thought stopping at home. In a calm moment, have your child practice saying, "No. Stop telling me that, worry brain. I can do this." When kids "talk back" to their worry brains and replace anxious thoughts with positive ones, they can interrupt the worry cycle and reset themselves.

Teach deep breathing:

Deep breathing is a great strategy for young children. Deep breathing slows down the heart rate and relieves muscle tension. Encourage your child to visualize blowing up a balloon while taking a very deep breath. Your child should inhale for a count of four, hold for four, and exhale for four.

The Stop, Think, Breathe app is an excellent resource for children with anxiety and ADHD. Through guided meditations and mindful breathing, kids learn to manage their anxious thoughts and replace negative/anxious thinking with calm/peaceful thinking.

Consider psychotherapy:

If your child's anxiety impacts his daily living (school, home, outside activities) and interferes with his ability to access the curriculum at school and enjoy his life, it's time to seek a licensed mental health professional. Through psychotherapy, kids can learn to manage their emotions and work through their triggers of stress and anxiety. Seek a referral for a child psychotherapist who specializes in anxiety for best results.

ADHD and Anxiety: What You Need to Know

At a Glance

Some of the challenges that come with ADHD can make kids anxious. Many kids with ADHD may have trouble managing emotions. Some kids may have an anxiety disorder as well as ADHD.

Anxiety is common in kids with ADHD. Many of the challenges that come with ADHD can make kids anxious. Kids with ADHD are also more likely to have an anxiety disorder than other kids.

It can be hard to tell whether a child has ADHD or anxiety because there's so much overlap in how they look in kids. Here's what you need to know about ADHD and anxiety—and what you can do to help your child.

The ADHD-Anxiety Connection

Kids with ADHD have trouble with executive functions. These are the skills that help us get organized, plan, manage time, and follow daily routines. Struggling with these skills day after day can be stressful. And chronic stress can lead to anxiety.

Kids with ADHD often have more trouble managing stress than kids who don't have ADHD, too. That's because ADHD affects how kids manage their emotions. Kids with ADHD may get so flooded with emotion that they have trouble thinking clearly about how to cope with the situation.

So, having ADHD can lead to anxiety. But kids with ADHD are also up to three times more likely to have an anxiety disorder than other kids. Because

ADHD and anxiety disorders often occur at the same time, some researchers think kids may be pre-wired to be both anxious and inattentive.

What an Anxious Child With ADHD May Look Like

Trouble managing emotions can affect kids' behavior in different ways. Some kids act up and draw attention to themselves. Others sit quietly and try not to be noticed. Here are some behaviors that may be signs of anxiety in a child with ADHD:

• Clowns around too much in class

• Seems irritable or argumentative

• Lies about schoolwork or other responsibilities that haven't been met

• Withdraws from people, maybe by retreating to the bedroom or bathroom

• Plays video games or watches TV non stop

Why Anxiety Is Sometimes Misdiagnosed as ADHD

Sometimes kids with anxiety can be misdiagnosed with ADHD, or vice versa. That's because on the surface, the two can look similar. Here are some of the ways kids with either may act—but for different reasons:

Have trouble paying attention. Kids with anxiety may seem tuned out or preoccupied, but they are really distracted by worries. Kids with ADHD are inattentive because of differences in the brain that affect focus.

Fidget constantly. Kids with anxiety may tap their foot nonstop during class because of nervous energy. Kids with ADHD fidget because of hyperactivity or trouble with impulse control.

Work slowly. Kids with anxiety may work slowly because they feel like they have to do something perfectly. Kids with ADHD take a long time to get things done because they have trouble starting tasks and focusing on them.

Don't turn in assignments. Kids with anxiety might get stuck on a task and be too anxious to ask for help. Kids with ADHD often don't turn in assignments because of poor planning skills and forgetfulness.

Struggle to make friends. Kids with social anxiety might be too fearful of social situations to make friends. Kids with ADHD might have trouble picking up on social cues because they struggle with focus. Or their impulsive behavior might annoy or alienate other kids.

There are lots of overlapping symptoms between ADHD and anxiety. But there are also key differences: Kids with anxiety disorders often show compulsive or perfectionist behavior. This isn't as common in kids with ADHD.

Kids with ADHD tend to struggle with organization. This isn't as common in kids with anxiety.

Kids with anxiety tend to worry more about socializing than kids with ADHD.

Kids with anxiety may also develop physical symptoms like sweaty palms, rapid breathing, and stomachaches.

How You Can Help

Get to know signs of anxiety in younger kids or teens and tweens, and take notes on what you see. Using an anxiety tracker can help you better understand when and why your child feels anxious.

Here are some other ways to help:

Tune in to your child's behavior. Try not to chalk them all up to ADHD. Acting up more than usual or disappearing into video games can be signs of anxiety. Ask if something is causing worry or uneasiness.

If your child talks about anxiety, validate those feelings. Rather than telling your child to "calm down," work together to figure out next steps to take.

Be mindful of your own anxiety. Some parents of anxious kids struggle with anxiety themselves. Remember that your child is learning how to respond to stressful situations by watching how you react to them. Kids often have an easier time coping with anxiety if their parents stay calm and positive.

Try not to take things personally. It can be upsetting when your child comes home from school and says something rude or offensive. But when kids do this, they're often letting off steam after a stressful day. When things have calmed down, brainstorm ways to decompress, like offering quiet time before you start asking about school.

Help your child see the big picture. If your child blows up when doing math homework, wait for things to calm down. Then encourage your child to reflect on what caused those feelings. Talk about what you both might be able to do next time to relieve some of that anxiety.

Consider outside help. If your child's anxiety gets in the way of functioning or enjoying life, talk to your health-care provider. If need be, they can refer you to a mental health professional who can help you and your child find the best path forward.

Keep in mind that getting a thorough evaluation is key to determining if your child has ADHD, an anxiety disorder, or both. This is especially important if you're considering medication. ADHD medication may relieve anxiety in some kids. But there's also a chance it may make some kids more anxious. It all depends on how sensitive a particular child's body is to a particular medication.

Anxiety can be a lifelong reality for some kids with ADHD. But with the right support, kids can manage both ADHD and anxiety, and thrive in school and in life.

Key Takeaways

Kids with ADHD are more likely to have anxiety than kids who don't have ADHD.

Sometimes kids with anxiety can be misdiagnosed with ADHD, or vice versa.

Keep track of signs of anxiety you see, and reach out to your health-care provider if you have concerns.

ADHD Adults

STRESS & ANXIETY

When Worry Begins to Paralyze You

"The genetic underpinnings of ADHD and anxiety overlap. They have a lot in common." Here, Dr. Ned Hallowell explains why you're so worried, and what to do about it.

A woman with ADHD showing signs of anxiety

Worry and anxiety often accompany attention deficit disorder (ADHD or ADD). So first, let's distinguish between the two. Worry has a target; one worries about something. Anxiety is usually free-floating, with no clear source or direction. Both are unpleasant, but anxiety may be more so, because the sufferer can't identify a cause.

Can Untreated ADD Cause Anxiety?

Worry and anxiety come with ADHD because attention deficit gives a person a lot to worry about. ADHD often leads a person astray, down blind alleys, or on wild goose chases. It causes a person to lose track of time and, suddenly, in a panic, get things done in an hour that might have taken a week. ADHD often induces a person to misspeak or to make an offensive or misleading remark without meaning to. In short, ADHD can turn a good day into chaos, a good week into mayhem, a good month into disaster, and a good life into one of missed chances and shattered hopes. A person with ADHD has a lot of trouble finding peace, harmony, or equanimity during the course of his life.

The genetic underpinnings of ADHD and anxiety overlap. I have treated people who suffer from worry and anxiety, as well as ADHD, for more than 30 years. They have a lot in common. Most worriers are creative and smart. It takes a lot of creativity and smarts to dream up all those things to worry about. I should know. I have ADHD and I am a worrier. People with ADHD live in a realm I call in my book, Worry: Hope and Help for a Common Condition, "the infinite web of 'what-if.'" We also tend to be creative, original, and come up with new ideas out of nowhere. I have come to believe we were born this way. Our genetic endowment gives us the reward of original thinking and the pain that comes when that thinking goes awry, as it sometimes does.

Worry and anxiety have an upside for the person who has ADHD. We are always searching for mental focus. The most riveting stimulus is physical pain. Put your finger near a flame, and you will pay attention to the flame. Worry and anxiety are the mental equivalent of physical pain. The person with ADHD may wake up and find that life is good. However, contentment is not riveting. So he scans the horizon looking for something to worry about. Once he finds an object of worry, it pierces his mind like a dagger. It becomes a source of focus throughout the day.

There are other sources of worry and anxiety, and both can bring on anxiety disorders, including phobias, generalized anxiety disorder (GAD), panic attacks, obsessive-compulsive disorder (OCD), post-traumatic stress disorder (PTSD), and more.

A little worry is healthy. We all need it. But when worry careens out of control, it is paralyzing. When worry paralyzes a person, it leads to loss of perspective, irrational thinking, and poor judgment. For full-blown anxiety disorders, one should consult a psychiatrist or other professional. But in the case of paralyzing worry, try the following three-step solution, which even children can be taught to use:

Treatment for the Symptoms of Anxiety Disorders

1. Never worry alone. Worrying alone leads a person to brood, globalize, awful-ize, and sink into a dark place. Talk with someone you like or love.

2. Get the facts. Paralyzing worry is usually rooted in wrong information, lack of information, or both. Don't take to heart everything you hear or read.

3. Make a plan. When you have a plan, you feel more in control and less vulnerable, which diminishes worry. If the plan doesn't work, revise it. That's what life is all about.

What's the Link Between Anxiety and ADHD

Attention deficit hyperactivity disorder (ADHD) and anxiety are separate conditions, but for a lot of folks they come as a package deal. About half of adults with ADHD also have anxiety disorder. If you're one of them, the right treatment can improve your ADHD symptoms and ease your anxious feelings, too.

What to Expect From ADHD and Anxiety

When you have anxiety along with ADHD, it may make some of your ADHD symptoms worse, such as feeling restless or having trouble concentrating. But anxiety disorder also comes with its own set of symptoms, like:

Constant worry about many different things

Feeling on edge

Stress

Fatigue

Trouble sleeping

Anxiety disorder is more than just having anxious feelings from time to time. It's a mental illness that can affect your relationships, work, and quality of life. Sometimes, anxiety comes as a result of ADHD. When that's the case, your worries are often about how much or how little you're able to get done. You're anxious about or overwhelmed by your ADHD.

When you have anxiety disorder on top of your ADHD, your worries are usually about a wide variety of things and not only tied to your ADHD struggles.

Talk to your doctor so the two of you can figure out where your anxiety is coming from. Some questions they may ask you are:

Do you worry about things that don't make sense?

Do you have a hard time controlling these worries?

Are you getting good sleep?

Are your fears and worries keeping you from doing your regular activities?

Do you feel anxious at least three to five times a week for an hour or more a day?

Have you had a big life event happen recently?

Do any of your family members have a history of anxiety?

How to Treat ADHD and Anxiety

To zero in on the best way to treat ADHD and anxiety, your doctor will likely look at which condition affects you the most. It's possible that your treatment for ADHD may ease your anxiety, so you may only need to take ADHD medication.

When you get treatment for ADHD, it can:

Cut your stress

Improve your attention so you manage tasks better

Give you mental energy to handle anxiety symptoms more easily

If your anxiety is a separate condition and not a symptom of ADHD, you may need to treat both disorders at the same time.

Some treatments can work for both ADHD and anxiety, such as:

• Cognitive behavioral therapy

• Relaxation techniques and meditation

• Prescription medications

Effects of ADHD Medication on Your Anxiety

The most common drugs that doctors suggest for ADHD are stimulants like methylphenidate and amphetamines. Even if you have anxiety, these meds may work well for your ADHD.

Anxiety is a common side effect of stimulants. Your doctor won't know how a medication will affect you until you take it, but it's possible stimulants may make your anxiety symptoms worse.

If that's the case for you, your doctor may suggest other medicines, such as the nonstimulant drug atomoxetine (Strattera).

Your doctor may also recommend antidepressants like:

• Bupropion (Wellbutrin)

• Desipramine (Norpramin)

• Imipramine (Tofranil)

• Nortriptyline (Pamelor)

• Venlafaxine (Effexor)

High blood pressure drugs like clonidine (Catapres, Kapvay) and guanfacine (Tenex, Intuniv) may also help.

How to treat kids with anxiety and ADHD

Medication and CBT usually are necessary for these highly impaired children.

Aaron, age 10, has been diagnosed with an anxiety disorder and attention-deficit/hyperactivity disorder (ADHD) but is not being treated with medication because his parents do not believe in psychopharmacology. They bring him to a specialized child anxiety clinic and ask for "urgent CBT" because his behavior at school is out of control.

Aaron rearranges the therapist's office furniture during much of the assessment interview. He also acknowledges many anxiety symptoms. The therapist doubts that cognitive-behavioral therapy (CBT) would help without other interventions.

Children with anxiety disorders and ADHD a common comorbid presentation—tend to be more impaired than those with either condition alone. Effective treatment usually requires for components including medication plus behavioral or cognitive-behavioral therapy. This article discusses clinical issues related to each component and describes how to successfully combine them into a treatment plan.

ADHD: attention-deficit/hyperactivity disorder

Medication options

Stimulants, atomoxetine, and selective serotonin reuptake inhibitors (SSRIs) have been advocated for children with anxiety and ADHD. Given the high risk of behavioral disinhibition with SSRIs in children, stimulants or atomoxetine are suggested as first-line medications.

Stimulants target ADHD symptoms primarily, but anxiety decreases in some children (24% in a recent trial) as ADHD symptoms are controlled. Because it is a selective norepinephrine reuptake inhibitor (SNRI), atomoxetine may target both ADHD and anxiety symptoms. When initiating these medications, "start low and go slow." Recommended dosing is no different for children with ADHD and anxiety than for those with ADHD alone.

Clinical Point

Atomoxetine may target both ADHD and anxiety symptoms, but improvements might not be evident for several weeks

Stimulant response rates for children with ADHD and anxiety vary among studies. Some report lower response rates than for children with ADHD alone and possibly more treatment-emergent side effects. The National Institute of Mental Health's Multimodal

Treatment Study of Children with ADHD (MTA) found that comorbid anxiety did not adversely affect behavioral response to stimulants but did moderate outcomes Adding intensive psychosocial intervention to stimulant treatment appeared to yield greater improvements in anxious children with ADHD, compared with stimulants alone.

Cognitive impairments related to inattention do not consistently improve with stimulant treatment. This is clinically important because children with ADHD and comorbid anxiety disorders can be very cognitively impaired.

Add an SSRI? Monotherapy is simpler and usually more acceptable to families, but a placebo-controlled study examined adding an SSRI (fluvoxamine) to methylphenidate treatment. Children with anxiety and ADHD who received adjunctive fluvoxamine did no better than those who received methylphenidate plus placebo.

Atomoxetine. A large, randomized, controlled trial of atomoxetine in this population found good tolerability and statistically significant reductions in ADHD and anxiety symptoms compared with placebo. Effect size was greater for ADHD symptoms than for anxiety symptoms, however, which supports smaller trials that show more consistent evidence of atomoxetine reducing ADHD symptoms than anxiety symptoms.

Similar to antidepressants with the SNRI chemical structure, atomoxetine's effectiveness for a given child takes several weeks to determine. This can be a problem in children who are highly distressed or impaired and require rapid symptomatic improvement.

Clinical Point

Consider individual CBT to reduce the distractions of group therapy, and seek a therapist who has experience working with this population

Recommendation. Consider a stimulant or atomoxetine initially for children with anxiety disorders and ADHD, and seek concurrent behavioral or cognitive-behavioral therapy. Caution families that: medication trial might be needed, as response may not be as consistent as in children with ADHD alone

medication-related improvements in ADHD symptoms will not necessarily be associated with reduced anxiety symptoms or improved academic ability

improvements with atomoxetine might not be evident for several weeks.

Medication dosing for children with ADHD
Expand table

Medication Recommended starting dosage Recommended maximum dosage 5 most common side effects in descending prevalence

Stimulants

Methylphenidate hydrochloride (Ritalin) 5 mg tid Total 60 mg/d Insomnia, nervousness, decreased appetite, dizziness, nausea

Methylphenidate hydrochloride (Concerta) 18 mg every morning 54 mg every morning Headache, abdominal pain, decreased appetite, vomiting, insomnia

Dextroamphetamine sulfate (Dexedrine) 5 mg every morning Total 40 mg/d Palpitations, restlessness, dizziness, dry mouth, decreased appetite

Mixed amphetamine salts (Adderall) 10 mg every morning 30 mg every morning Decreased appetite, insomnia, abdominal pain, emotional lability, vomiting

Nonstimulant

Atomoxetine (Strattera) 0.5 mg/kg/d 1.2 mg/kg/d

ADHD and anxiety: What's the connection?

The connection between ADHD and anxiety Signs and symptoms of co-existing anxiety and ADHD Treating both anxiety and ADHD

Attention deficit hyperactivity disorder and anxiety disorders frequently occur together. These conditions can simply exist simultaneously, or ADHD may contribute to the development of the anxiety disorder.

Individuals with ADHD often have other mental health conditions. In fact, around half of adults with ADHD also have an anxiety disorder.

Sometimes, symptoms can be difficult to tell apart from one another as they share certain symptoms. For instance, in both anxiety disorders and ADHD, the individual may have difficulty concentrating or relaxing.

Learning about the differences between the two disorders is important in the management and treatment of both. Anxiety can significantly impact how someone with ADHD manages their condition.

The connection between ADHD and anxiety

ADHD often begins in childhood.

Attention deficit hyperactivity disorder (ADHD) usually begins during childhood, and can continue to adulthood in some people. This developmental disorder is typically associated with symptoms such as:

a short attention span

fidgeting

hyperactivity

impulsivity

restlessness

According to the Anxiety and Depression Association of America, approximately 50 percent of American adults with ADHD also have an anxiety disorder. The National Resource Centre on ADHD estimate that up to 30 percent of children with the condition experience anxiety.

Currently, it is unclear why anxiety and ADHD appear together so frequently. Factors such as genetics, premature birth, and environmental toxins are thought to play a part in ADHD, so it is possible that they also influence anxiety disorders; more research is needed.

A person with an anxiety disorder is likely to experience long-lasting feelings of nervousness, fear, and worry. Although occasional anxiety is normal, those with anxiety disorders experience anxiety most, or all, of the time.

They may have difficulty identifying and controlling their specific fears and worries. These feelings tend to be out of proportion to the situation, and can interfere with people's daily lives and relationships with others.

There are many types of anxiety disorders, including generalized anxiety disorder (GAD), panic disorder, and social anxiety disorder.

The connection

Although anxiety and ADHD may occur together, ADHD is not an anxiety disorder.

Sometimes, anxiety can occur independently of ADHD. Other times, it can be as a result of living with ADHD.A person who has ADHD and misses a work deadline or forgets to study for an important exam can become stressed and worried. Even the fear of forgetting to do such important tasks may cause them anxiety.

If these feelings and situations continue, which they do for many people with ADHD, they can lead to an anxiety disorder.

Furthermore, the medications used to treat ADHD, especially stimulant medications such as amphetamines, can cause symptoms of anxiety. Genetics may also play a role.

Signs and symptoms of co-existing anxiety and ADHD

It can be difficult to differentiate between anxiety and ADHD as the two conditions can appear similar. Some signs and symptoms that are common to both conditions include:

difficulty socializing

fidgeting

inattentiveness

working slowly or failing to complete work on time

According to Understood, additional signs of anxiety in children with ADHD can include:

being irritable or argumentative

causing trouble in class

playing video games or watching TV most of the time

telling lies about schoolwork or other responsibilities that haven't been completed

withdrawing from people

How to tell the difference

Although there are many things in common, there are some differences between the two conditions. Anxiety is primarily a disorder of nervousness, worry, and fear, while ADHD is characterized by a lack of attention and focus. People with anxiety can also display compulsive or perfectionist behaviors, which aren't typically seen in those with ADHD.

Someone with an anxiety disorder will find it difficult to concentrate during certain situations that cause them to feel anxious. However, someone with ADHD will find it difficult to concentrate most or all of the time.

Although friends and family may recognize the symptoms of anxiety, ADHD, or both, a health professional should carry out a full evaluation before a diagnosis is made.

Treating both anxiety and ADHD

When anxiety and ADHD occur together, they can make daily activities more difficult. A person with ADHD who also has anxiety may find concentrating on tasks even more challenging. Therefore, it is very important to get proper treatment to ensure a better quality of life.

Anxiety can also complicate ADHD treatment because it tends to make people afraid to try new things. And, to deal with ADHD, new strategies might need to be employed to keep on top of the condition.

Treatment plans will vary based on the individual and the situation. Some people may benefit from having both conditions treated simultaneously.

Other times, treating just one of the conditions might be the priority. This may be appropriate if ADHD is the cause of the anxiety, as treating the ADHD can reduce the anxiety.

There are many different treatment options available to those with both ADHD and anxiety.

Medication

Prescription medications are most commonly used in treating ADHD. However, if stimulant medications are causing symptoms of anxiety, other nonstimulant medications may be prescribed. Anti-anxiety medications might also be considered.

If taking several medications is not recommended, or if the person does not wish to take them, a doctor may prescribe medication for one of the disorders and treat the other with therapeutic or lifestyle interventions.

Therapy and relaxation techniques

The anxiety related to ADHD may be better managed with:

Cognitive behavioral therapy (CBT): this short-term intervention helps people to change their thinking patterns in order to positively influence their behavior. CBT is widely used for anxiety disorders, and has been shown to be effective in the treatment of GAD and many other conditions.

Relaxation techniques: practicing techniques, such as meditation, progressive muscle relaxation, visualization, and deep-breathing exercises can help treat stress and anxiety by slowing the heart rate, reducing muscle tension, and boosting concentration and mood.

Lifestyle changes

[Woman getting some sleep]

Having a regular sleep cycle can help reduce symptoms of anxiety.

In addition to taking medication, considering therapy, and practicing relaxation techniques, several lifestyle factors can help those with anxiety related to ADHD.

Sleep: tiredness can worsen feelings of anxiety. At least one study has indicated that anxiety in children with ADHD is linked with sleep disturbances.

People should aim to go to sleep and wake up at the same time each day.

Those who struggle to fall asleep or stay asleep should discuss the issue with their doctor.

Exercise: regular exercise can reduce anxiety in a number of ways, including through the release of brain chemicals that boost mood.

Schedule tasks: keeping a list of tasks and activities that need to be completed, and setting realistic timeframes for each, can ensure goals are remembered and achieved. This can help reduce anxiety levels.

Nutrition: eating healthful and balanced meals and staying hydrated can help manage anxiety. Reducing the intake of caffeine and alcohol may also be useful, as both of these interfere with sleeping patterns.

Try to give the doctor as much information as possible on the symptoms experienced by the person in their care, even those that do not seem related to ADHD or anxiety. This will help the doctor to make an accurate diagnosis and create an effective treatment plan.

Be patient. Anxiety can cause people to become afraid to try new things, including new treatments for ADHD or the anxiety itself. Feeling anxious can also add to the lack of focus and forgetfulness experienced by those with ADHD.

Be supportive. Being critical or negative will only add to the stress and worry experienced by those with ADHD and anxiety.

Control parental anxiety. Children learn to respond to situations based on their parents' reactions. Parents of children with ADHD who remain calm and positive will influence their children to do the same in stressful situations.

Consider parenting skills training. Parents can learn new ways of understanding and responding to children with ADHD.

Consider family therapy. This may be useful for parents and siblings who need additional support in dealing with the challenges of living with someone with ADHD.

Made in the USA
Columbia, SC
06 February 2026

78887184R00049